Dive into Wellness

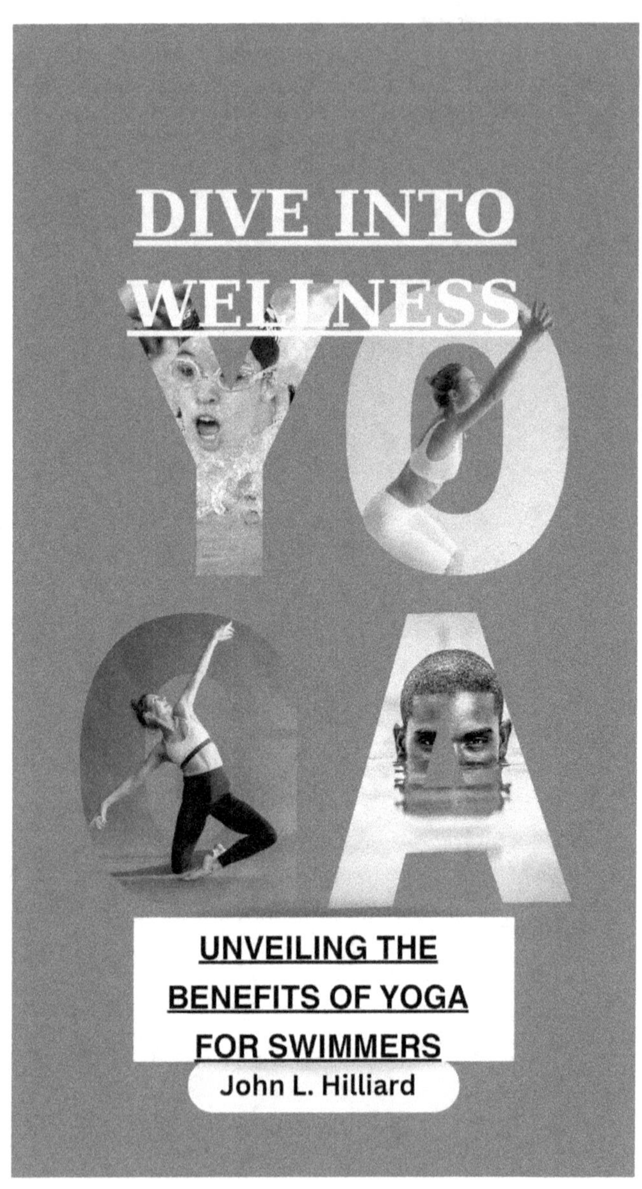

DIVE INTO
WELLNESS
YOGA
UNVEILING THE
BENEFITS OF YOGA
FOR SWIMMERS
John L. Hilliard

Unveiling the Benefits of Yoga for Swimmers

John L. Hilliard

Table of content

Introduction:

Adding yoga to a swimmer's regimen creates a potent synergy in the fluid world of swimming, where every stroke is a ballet with the water. Past the edge of the water, the mat calls, providing a comprehensive method to improve mental toughness in addition to physical strength. Let's explore the many advantages of yoga for swimmers and explore the world where buoyancy and breath collide.

Range of Motion and Flexibility: Yoga's mild asanas and stretches promote range of motion, which helps swimmers become more flexible. Improved flexibility helps to maintain a fluid and effective swimming technique by improving stroke refinement and injury prevention.

Strength and Core Stability: Yoga and swimming together provide a strong base. Yoga positions that focus on strengthening the core are especially beneficial for developing the stabilizing muscles needed for accurate swimming. A stronger core contributes to better balance and body control, which makes swimming more fluid.

Breath Control and Lung Capacity: The breath is the foundation of both swimming and yoga. Yoga techniques enable swimmers to seamlessly synchronize breath and movement because they place a strong emphasis on mindful breathing. This timing maximizes oxygen uptake and increases lung capacity, giving swimmers a higher threshold for endurance.

Injury Prevention and Rehabilitation: Yoga's low-impact qualities work well with swimming's high-impact requirements, protecting against injuries. Furthermore, yoga provides a mild yet efficient form of therapy for swimmers who are recovering, helping them restore their muscle and flexibility.

Reducing Stress and Improving Mental Health:

Yoga's meditative techniques are an ally to swimming's healing properties. Yoga's contemplative elements help to reduce stress and ease the mental strain that comes with rigorous training. Not only does a healthy mind improve performance, but it also fosters a positive outlook on the challenging world of professional swimming.

Enhancement of Balance: In yoga, balancing poses act as a sort of bridge between the water and the mat. Swimmers develop stability and control by learning the skill of balance, both mentally and physically. This improved balance not only keeps the swimmer from falling on land, but it also makes it easier for them to gracefully maneuver through currents and waves.

Community and Mental Resilience: Yoga is a group practice that takes place outside of the studio; it's not only a lonely endeavor. The sense of camaraderie and mental resilience that yoga sessions build is beneficial for swimmers. The mindset of the swimmer is strengthened by sharing the struggles and victories on the mat, forming a network of support that extends beyond the pool.

Flexibility in Changing Conditions: Yoga instills flexibility, which is a crucial skill for swimmers dealing with erratic water conditions. The mental toughness that swimmers develop on the mat prepares them to face obstacles head-on, whether they are unfavorable weather, powerful currents, or unanticipated competitive dynamics. Yoga turns into a practice for accepting change with composure and concentration.

Warm-Up Exercises Before the Swim to Improve Your Performance

Start by slowly turning your neck in both clockwise and counterclockwise directions. This easy-to-do warm-up helps your neck muscles become more flexible and relaxed so they're ready for the rhythmic movements of swimming.

Arm Swings: Use active arm swings to loosen up your arms and shoulders. Maintain a straight stance and move your arms in a deliberate forward and backward motion. This enhances range of motion and promotes the blood flow to the shoulder joints, both of which are important for strong strokes.

Torso Twists: Include torso twists in your warm-up exercises to strengthen your core. Place your feet shoulder-width apart, then turn your upper body in a circular motion. In addition to warming up your spine, this motion improves your body's ability to rotate, which is crucial for effective swimming strokes.

Leg Swings: Use leg swings to get your lower body ready for the resistance of the water. Swing one leg controlled forward and backward while holding onto a solid surface. This dynamic stretch prepares your legs for the forceful kicks you'll execute during your swim by focusing on the hamstrings, quadriceps, and hip flexors.

Ankle Rolls: The ankles are crucial to swimming yet are frequently disregarded. Lifting one foot off the floor and rotating your ankle in a circular motion is how you perform ankle rolls. This helps to warm up the ankle joints, which is important for giving a powerful push-off when starting and turning.

Deep Breathing: Use deep breathing techniques to help you into a focused mental state. Breathe in deeply through your nose, letting the breath fill your lungs, and then gently release the air through your mouth. This exercise increases oxygen intake and promotes mental calmness, which prepares the body and mind for a concentrated and easy swim.

Incorporate dynamic stretches to work on your main muscle groups. Arm circles, leg lunges, and high knees all serve to increase circulation, loosen up the muscles in your body that you'll be using when swimming. Better performance is facilitated by dynamic stretching, which prepares your body for the dynamic movements of swimming.

Practice your water entry by acting out a smooth entry before you actually step into the water. As you stand at the pool's edge, picture your dive and practice dipping in with little splash. This helps you become more proficient and prepares your body for the first shock, so you can move smoothly from the pool to the water.

Visualization Technique: Set aside some time to visualize yourself mentally. Imagine yourself making flawless strokes and floating through the water with ease. Gaining confidence and improving muscle memory through visualization gives you a mental advantage when you enter the water.

Running in Place: Running in place causes your body temperature to rise and your heart rate to increase. Your cardiovascular system is stimulated by this easy aerobic activity, which makes sure your body is sufficiently warmed up for the demands of swimming. For a few minutes, jogging nevertheless can help improve joint mobility.

Shoulder Rotations: Use deliberate rotations to concentrate on your shoulder joints. To improve your flexibility and range of motion, make both circles with your shoulders. As the shoulders are widely used in many strokes, this is especially advantageous for swimmers. A proper warm-up for your shoulders reduces the possibility of strain and damage during swimming.

Calf Raises: These exercises will strengthen your lower legs and improve the stability of your ankles. Lift your heels off the ground and rise onto the balls of your feet while maintaining a hip-width distance between your feet. This workout helps build the strength required for strong kicks in the water in addition to warming up your calf muscles.

Stretches that Are Dynamic and Help Your Body Get Ready for Swimming

Arm Circles: Extend your arms straight out to the sides while keeping your feet shoulder-width apart. Start with little circles with your arms and work your way up to larger ones. This dynamic stretch enhances range of motion and loosens up the shoulders, both of which are necessary for strong strokes.

Leg Swings: Controllably swing one leg forward and backward while holding onto a stable surface, such as the edge of the pool. This dynamic stretch works the hamstrings and hip flexors, increasing the flexibility needed for effective kicking and fluid swimming motion.

Torso Twists: Place your feet shoulder-width apart and stand straight. As you slowly rotate your torso to one side and then the other, your arms should follow suit. This stretch works the core, improving flexibility in rotation, which is important for arranging the body correctly during strokes.

High Knees: Make a marching motion with your knees lifted toward your chest while you remain in position. This vigorous stretch warms up your hip flexors, quickens your pulse rate, and prepares your lower body for the demands of such movement.

Dynamic Torso Bend: Place your arms high and your feet shoulder-width apart. Reaching toward your knee, bend at the waist to one side, then switch to the other side with ease. This stretch helps with body roll during freestyle and backstroke strokes by enhancing lateral flexibility.

Calf Raises: Locate a stable platform to place your heels on and raise them off the ground so that you are standing on your balls of feet. To warm up your lower leg muscles, carefully elevate your calves. This stretch helps you execute strong push-offs and kicks off the pool floor.

Swimmer's Shoulder Opener: Raise your arms slightly and straighten them while arranging your fingers behind your back. To achieve the best arm extension during strokes, this stretch opens up the shoulders and chest. Additionally, it helps shield swimmers' shoulders from common accidents.

Butterfly Stretch: Sit with your knees bent outward and your soles together. Gently press your knees toward the floor while using your hands to hold your feet. The inner thighs and hip flexors, which are essential for the smooth leg motions in breaststroke, are the focus of this stretch.

Rotate your wrists in a circular motion while extending your arms in front of you. For swimmers in particular, this stretch is helpful because it increases wrist flexibility, which is necessary for performing effective hand movements and stroke entrance.

Core Activation Plank: Lie down on your back with your head and heels in a straight line. Hold the pose for 20–30 seconds to contract your core muscles. Stability and balance in the water are facilitated by this dynamic exercise that engages the core.

Dynamic Back Arch: Arc your back while extending your arms overhead while standing with your feet hip-width apart. This stretch targets the spine, increasing range of motion and flexibility to facilitate more fluid and deliberate backstroke motions.

Inhale Control Exercise: Take a deep inhale through your nose and gently release it through your mouth to practice controlled breathing. In addition to reducing anxiety, this exercise gets your breathing regular while swimming, which maximizes oxygen uptake and energy conservation.

The Benefits of Concentrated Breathing Methods

Stroke Synchronization: In aquatic ballet, stroke synchronization is essential. Concentrated breathing flows in unison with every stroke, forming a beautiful ballet between the swimmer's motions and breath patterns. Because of this synchronization, resistance is reduced, resulting in more fluid, effective strokes and improved water glide.

Oxygen Optimization: Think of oxygen as the premium gasoline and your lungs as fuel tanks. Breathing deliberately increases the amount of oxygen that reaches the muscles, preventing weariness from setting in. Swimmers maximize oxygen usage by timing their intake and release of air, which increases their endurance and pushes the limits of their performance.

Mental Clearance and Calm: Concentrated breathing serves as a lighthouse for mental clarity and calmness amidst the steady waves. In addition to providing the body with oxygen, deep, slow breaths act as a meditative anchor, helping the mind become clear-headed and peaceful. This mental clarity boosts confidence and improves overall performance, making it the secret weapon against anxiety.

Developing Resilience: Just like any other activity, swimming requires resilience. Resilience is cultivated by focused breathing, which teaches swimmers how to overcome obstacles underwater and adjust to changing circumstances. In choppy conditions, the swimmer's capacity to maintain composure and resilience in the face of difficulty is reinforced by the controlled breath, which acts as a lifeline.

Better Body Position and Buoyancy: Visualize your breath as a buoyant energy that lifts you through the water with ease. Concentrated breathing helps swimmers maintain the best possible body alignment by improving buoyancy. This improves hydrodynamics and lowers drag, increasing stroke efficiency and encouraging a smooth glide.

Enhanced Recovery: In swimming, recuperation is just as important as propulsion. During the recovery phase, focused breathing is essential for swimmers to quickly restore their oxygen levels. Effective exhalation guarantees that carbon dioxide is released, preventing its accumulation and promoting a faster recovery period in between strokes.

Strategic Pacing: Swimming athletes who have mastered focused breathing are equipped with a tactical tool for timing. Athletes can adjust their breathing to meet the demands of various swimming techniques and race distances by varying the rhythm and depth of their breaths. Even in the longest races, swimmers may sustain peak energy levels thanks to this tactical technique, which guarantees a good finish.

Overcoming Anxiety and Developing Confidence: For inexperienced swimmers in particular, the water may be both alluring and frightening. Concentrated breathing is an effective tool for conquering anxiety and turns water into a calming substance. Swimmers develop confidence, overcome phobias, and realize their full potential through deliberate breathing exercises.

Injury Prevention: Although swimming is a low-impact activity, accidents can still happen. Through the promotion of a balanced distribution of effort across muscle groups, focused breathing helps to prevent injuries. By encouraging a smoother, more regulated range of motion, proper breathing practices lower the danger of strains or injuries that are frequently linked to uncontrolled movements.

Lifelong Wellness: Concentrated breathing has several advantages that go well beyond the pool's lanes. Swimmers develop a practice that goes beyond competing objectives when they incorporate these strategies into their routines. Concentrated breathing becomes an essential component of long-term health, providing enhanced cardiovascular health, stress reduction, and a contemplative haven that goes far beyond the shore.

After-Swim Recovery Positions

Child's Pose (Balasana): Start your healing process with this mild yoga pose. This pose helps you to relax by lengthening your spine, stretching your hips, and relieving tension in your neck and shoulders.

Thread the Needle Pose (Parsva Balasana): This pose helps release tension in the upper back and shoulders. This position encourages flexibility and eases any stiffness brought on the swimming strokes by offering a deep stretch for the upper back and shoulders.

Cobra Pose (Bhujangasana): This pose opens up the chest and strengthens the spine. This backbend helps release tension in the lower back and counteracts the forward motion of swimming. To maximize the relaxing effect, concentrate on taking deliberate breaths.

Adho Mukha Svanasana (Downward Facing Dog): To extend your entire body, transition into this pose. This pose works the shoulders, calves, and hamstrings, giving the muscles used in swimming a complete release. Savor the upside-down posture to improve blood flow and lessen exhaustion.

Legs Up the Wall Pose (Viparita Karani): This pose improves circulation and rejuvenates the legs. This healing inversion aids in removing extra fluid from the legs, which lowers swelling and speeds up healing. This is a great stance to help you relax and reap the advantages of your swim.

Seated Forward Bend (Paschimottanasana): Conclude your post-swim warm-up with this pose. This position promotes flexibility and releases any remaining tension by stretching the entire back of your body, from your calves to your spine. To further relax, pay attention to your breathing.

End your post-swim recovery session with the ultimate relaxation pose, Corpse Pose (Savasana). Allow your body to thoroughly assimilate the advantages of the preceding poses as you lie on your back. Pay attention to relaxing the body and mind, letting go of any last bits of tension, and accepting a deeply relaxed condition. Savasana offers a vital chance to combine the mental and physical facets of your healing.

Breathing Exercises: Use attentive breathing techniques to enhance your recovery poses.

Breathe diaphragmatically to increase oxygenation and induce relaxation. Breathing deliberately and slowly can help lower stress, expand lung capacity, and speed up your body's healing process.

Nutrition and Hydration: Make sure you eat foods high in nutrients and stay properly hydrated to aid in your body's healing. Restore electrolytes that you lost during swimming and provide your muscles the nutrition they need to heal. An optimally composed post-swim snack, including a blend of carbohydrates and protein, can facilitate recuperation and resupply of energy.

Self-Massage: Use massage balls or foam rollers to finish off your post-swim recovery regimen. Apply little pressure to tense or sore areas of muscle to help loosen knots and increase blood flow. Self-massage speeds up the healing process and helps to release tense muscles.

Relaxation Poses to Release Tension in Swimming

Floatation Meditation:

Begin by floating on your back, allowing the water to cradle you.Shut your eyes and pay attention to your breathing.Inhale deeply, feeling your chest rise, and exhale slowly, letting go of any stress. The gentle support of the water promotes relaxation, creating a serene environment for mental repose.

Water-Embrace Stretch:

While standing in chest-deep water, extend your arms outward and slowly rotate your wrists in circular motions. Feel the resistance of the water against your movements, stretching your arms and shoulders. This pose enhances flexibility and relieves tension in the upper body, leaving you feeling more fluid in the water.

Seahorse Pose:

For a soothing lower back stretch, lie on your stomach in the water, arms extended in front. Slowly lift one leg at a time, engaging your glutes and lower back muscles. This pose not only eases tension but also strengthens your core, contributing to better body balance in the water.

Zen Flutter Kick:

While floating on your back, initiate a gentle flutter kick with your legs. Allow the water's resistance to guide your movements, focusing on the rhythmic pattern. This mindful flutter kick not only works your leg muscles but also serves as a moving meditation, calming the mind and fostering a sense of tranquility.

Buoyancy Bliss:

Utilize a buoyancy aid to support your body in a relaxed, horizontal position. Close your eyes and let the water cradle you. Allow the gentle rocking of the water to massage away tension. This pose promotes a meditative state, making it an ideal conclusion to your swimming session.

Sunset Surrender Savasana:

Float on your back, allowing the water to support your entire body. Extend your arms and legs comfortably, mimicking the classic yoga Savasana pose. Close your eyes and focus on the sensation of weightlessness. As you surrender to the water's embrace, visualize a peaceful sunset, letting the colors wash away any lingering tension. This pose encourages full-body relaxation and a mental escape from the demands of daily life.

Coral Rejuvenation Twist:

Stand in chest-deep water and gently twist your torso to one side, reaching your arm across your body. Feel the stretch along your spine and engage your core. Hold the position for a few breaths, then switch to the other side. This twisting pose promotes spinal flexibility, releasing tension accumulated during the day, and enhancing your overall swimming experience.

Moonlit Mindful Breaststroke:

Transition into a slow and deliberate breaststroke, focusing on the fluidity of your movements. Emphasize the stretch in your arms and legs as you glide through the water. Consciously breathe in sync with your strokes, allowing the rhythmic pattern to create a meditative state. This mindful approach to swimming not only enhances your technique but also clears your mind of stressors.

Reef Reflection Visualization:

As you float in a relaxed position, imagine yourself surrounded by a vibrant coral reef. Envision the colorful fish gracefully swimming by and the gentle sway of underwater plants. This visualization technique helps shift your focus away from stressors, promoting mental clarity and relaxation. Combine it with slow, deep breaths for a truly immersive experience.

Submerge yourself in shoulder-deep water and perform slow, deliberate arm movements, creating resistance against the water. This hydrotherapy-inspired pose promotes joint flexibility and alleviates tension in the shoulders and arms. Embrace the soothing sensation of water enveloping you, turning your swim into a therapeutic journey for both body and mind.

Gentle Stretches for Muscles in Motion

Neck Rotations:

Begin your routine with slow and controlled neck rotations. Gently tilting your head from side to side and rotating it in circular motions helps alleviate tension in the neck and upper back—a common area of strain during repetitive swimming motions.

Shoulder Rolls:

Swimming heavily relies on shoulder strength and flexibility. Perform backward and forward shoulder rolls to warm up and loosen the muscles surrounding the shoulders. This prepares your body for the freestyle, breaststroke, and butterfly strokes.

Triceps Stretch:

Extend one arm overhead and reach down your back, gently patting yourself on the back with your other hand. This triceps stretch targets the muscles used in the powerful pull phase of each stroke, promoting better extension and reducing the risk of overuse injuries.

Chest Opener:

Counteract the forward motion of swimming by incorporating a chest opener stretch. Clasp your hands behind your back and straighten your arms, opening up your chest. This stretch improves posture and flexibility, essential for a streamlined and efficient swim.

Hip Flexor Stretch:

Strengthen your kicking abilities by focusing on your hip flexors. Kneel on one knee with the other foot in front, leaning slightly forward. This stretch helps alleviate tightness in the hip flexors, crucial for a powerful and effective kick in various swimming strokes.

Quadriceps Stretch:

Swimming engages the entire body, including the quadriceps. Stand on one leg, grab your ankle, and gently pull your heel towards your buttocks. This stretch enhances flexibility in the quads, aiding in smoother leg movements during kicks and turns.

Ankle Flexibility Exercises:

Optimize your flutter and dolphin kicks by incorporating ankle flexibility exercises. Point and flex your feet, trace circles with your toes, and perform toe taps to increase the range of motion in your ankles, facilitating more fluid and powerful kicks.

Back Stretch:

A supple and strong back is fundamental for a streamlined swim. While seated, extend your legs in front of you and reach forward, aiming to touch your toes. This back stretch not only targets the lower back but also enhances the flexibility of the entire spine, contributing to a smoother and more controlled swim.

Butterfly Stretch:

Embrace the graceful beauty of the butterfly stroke by incorporating a dedicated stretch. Sitting with the soles of your feet together, gently press your knees toward the ground. This stretch opens up the hips and improves the range of motion needed for the rhythmic butterfly kick.

Hamstring Stretch:

Sit on the pool deck or a mat with one leg extended straight and the other bent, foot against the inner thigh. Reach forward toward your toes, feeling the stretch in your hamstrings. Flexible hamstrings are essential for efficient kicks and proper body positioning in the water.

Calf Stretch:

Enhance ankle flexibility and alleviate tension in the calves with a simple calf stretch. Stand facing a wall, place your hands on it, and step one foot back, keeping it straight. Bend the front knee while pressing the back heel into the floor. Switch legs to ensure both calves receive equal attention.

Core Rotation:

Improve the rotational aspect of your strokes by incorporating a seated core rotation stretch. Sit with your legs extended, twist your torso to one side, placing your opposite elbow outside the bent knee. This stretch targets the core muscles crucial for stability and balance during various swimming movements.

Power of Balance and Core Strength in Swimming

Balancing Act:

Achieving equilibrium in the water is akin to mastering the delicate dance of weight distribution. Balanced body position minimizes drag, allowing swimmers to glide effortlessly through each stroke. Whether executing a streamlined dive or maintaining poise during a flip turn, a swimmer's ability to harmonize body movements with water resistance is pivotal.

Core Strength as the Propeller:

The core, often referred to as the body's powerhouse, serves as the propeller driving every stroke. From freestyle to butterfly, a strong core not only generates force but also stabilizes the body, enhancing control and precision. Engaging the core muscles optimally transforms swimmers into aquatic dynamos, enabling them to propel through the water with maximum efficiency.

Streamlined Speed:

Picture a streamlined torpedo cutting through the water – that's the result of a finely tuned balance and a robust core. When a swimmer maintains a hydrodynamic posture, drag is minimized, allowing for increased speed and reduced energy expenditure. The quest for streamlined perfection is an ongoing journey that separates the good from the exceptional in the world of competitive swimming.

Turning the Tide with Core Stability:

Turns and transitions are the heartbeat of any swim race. A powerful core provides the stability needed for swift and precise turns, ensuring minimal loss of momentum. Swimmers with a well-conditioned core can seamlessly navigate the fluid dynamics of turns, gaining a crucial advantage over competitors.

Preventing Injury, Enhancing Endurance:

Beyond performance, the benefits extend to injury prevention and endurance. A balanced body and strong core contribute to improved body alignment, reducing the risk of strain and injury. Moreover, endurance is amplified as the core muscles act as a reservoir of strength, allowing swimmers to sustain optimal performance over longer distances.

Masterful Poses for Superior Stability and Balance

The Streamlined Torpedo:

Pose: Extend your body in a straight line, arms clasped overhead, with your head aligned between your arms.

Benefits: Improves hydrodynamics, minimizes drag, and enhances overall body alignment, fostering stability and balance.

The Flutter Kick Perfection:

Pose: Lay on your back, arms at your sides, and execute a flutter kick with pointed toes.

Benefits: Strengthens core muscles, refines leg movement, and promotes stability by engaging the entire body in a synchronized motion.

The Precision Plank:

Pose: Assume a plank position with your forearms on the water surface, keeping your body parallel to the water.

Benefits: Builds core strength, stabilizes the body, and enhances balance by training the muscles that support streamlined swimming.

The Controlled Buoyancy Backstroke:

Pose: Float on your back, arms extended, and perform a controlled flutter kick.

Benefits: Enhances balance by focusing on leg movement while allowing you to refine your backstroke technique with improved body positioning.

The Dynamic Dolphin Dive:

Pose: Emulate a dolphin dive by pushing off the pool wall, arms stretched forward, and body streamlined.

Benefits: Develops core strength, refines diving technique, and hones stability by navigating smoothly through the water.

The Taut Tuck:

Pose: Curl into a tight tuck position while executing a quick rotation, then extend into a streamlined position.

Benefits: Sharpens agility, refines rotational movements, and improves balance through controlled transitions.

The Zen Zenith Float:

Pose: Float on your back with arms extended and legs relaxed, allowing your body to find a state of serene equilibrium.

Benefits: Promotes relaxation, mindfulness, and a heightened sense of body awareness, essential for maintaining stability during prolonged swims.

The Cross-Connect Twist:

Pose: Engage in a horizontal cross position, twisting your upper body and kicking rhythmically to each side.

Benefits: Enhances rotational flexibility, strengthens oblique muscles, and improves balance by challenging your body to adapt to changing directions.

The Supine Stability Stretch:

Pose: Float on your stomach, arms extended forward, and legs relaxed, focusing on elongating your body.

Benefits: Encourages flexibility, lengthens the spine, and reinforces stability by promoting a streamlined posture in the water.

The Meditative Breaststroke Glide:

Pose: Transition smoothly between breaststroke kicks and gliding, focusing on a slow, controlled rhythm.

Benefits: Improves coordination, refines breaststroke technique, and fosters stability through deliberate movements and rhythmic breathing.

The Buoyant Butterfly Challenge:

Pose: Practice the butterfly stroke with an emphasis on maintaining a consistent and controlled undulating motion.

Benefits: Strengthens the core and shoulders, refines butterfly technique, and challenges balance through the unique combination of powerful strokes.

The Side-Plank Swivel:

Pose: Execute a side plank in the water, lifting one arm toward the sky and rotating your torso in a controlled manner.

Benefits: Targets lateral stability, strengthens the core, and enhances balance by engaging muscles on one side of the body at a time.

Core-Strengthening Asanas for Swimmers

Plank Pose (Kumbhakasana):

Description: Begin in a push-up position, arms straight, and hold your body parallel to the ground.

Benefits: Engages the entire core, improves balance, and stabilizes the spine—essential for streamlined swimming.

Boat Pose (Navasana):

Description: Sit on the floor, lift your legs, and balance on your sit bones, forming a V shape with your body.

Benefits: Strengthens the abdominal muscles, hip flexors, and spine, promoting better body control during strokes.

Dolphin Pose (Svanasana, Makara Adho Mukha):

Description: From a plank position, lower your forearms to the ground, forming a straight line from head to heels.

Benefits: Targets the core, shoulders, and back, enhancing overall endurance for long-distance swims.

Bridge Pose (Setu Bandhasana):

Description: Lie on your back, bend your knees, and lift your hips towards the ceiling.

Benefits: Activates the core, glutes, and lower back, fostering a powerful kick and improved body alignment in the water.

The Parrot Lunge, or Parrotta Anjaneyasana:

Description: From a lunge position, twist your torso towards the front knee, maintaining a strong and stable stance.

Benefits: Increases rotational flexibility, a key element for efficient turns and strokes in swimming.

Supine Spinal Twist (Supta Matsyendrasana):

Description: Lie on your back, bring your knee across your body, and twist your torso in the opposite direction.

Benefits: Releases tension in the spine, enhances flexibility, and aids in developing a smoother, more streamlined swim.

Upward Plank Pose (Purvottanasana):

Description: Sit with legs extended, place hands behind you, lift hips towards the ceiling, creating a straight line from head to heels.

Benefits: Targets the core, shoulders, and arms, contributing to a powerful push-off from the pool wall and improved upper body strength.

Warrior III (Virabhadrasana III):

Description: Stand on one leg, extend the other leg behind you, and reach arms forward, forming a straight line from head to heel.

Benefits: Develops core strength, balance, and concentration—essential for stability and control during various swimming strokes.

Cobra Pose (Bhujangasana):

Description: Lie on your stomach, place palms beside your chest, and lift your upper body, keeping your lower body grounded.

Benefits: Strengthens the entire back, opens the chest, and enhances spine flexibility, contributing to a more efficient swim posture.

Seated Forward Bend (Paschimottanasana):

Description: Sit with legs extended, hinge at the hips, and reach towards your toes, keepin your back straight.

Benefits: Stretches the hamstrings, lower back, and shoulders, promoting flexibility crucial for streamlined body positioning in the water.

The Crucial Role of Flexibility for Swimmers

The Foundation of Fluidity:

Flexibility is the cornerstone of fluid and efficient swimming movements. Swimmers with increased flexibility experience improved range of motion, allowing for longer and more powerful strokes. A well-rounded flexibility routine enhances joint mobility, enabling swimmers to achieve optimal body positioning throughout each stroke. This foundation of fluidity not only reduces resistance in the water but also minimizes the risk of injury, paving the way for consistent, high-level performance.

Stroke-Specific Flexibility:

Different strokes demand distinct ranges of motion, emphasizing the importance of stroke-specific flexibility. Freestyle requires a supple rotation of the torso, while butterfly demands exceptional shoulder flexibility. Breaststroke and backstroke rely heavily on the flexibility of the hips and ankles. By tailoring flexibility exercises to match the requirements of each stroke, swimmers can fine-tune their bodies to meet the nuanced demands of their chosen discipline.

Improved Healing and Injury Avoidance:

Flexibility training isn't solely about reaching extreme positions; it plays a crucial role in recovery and injury prevention. Engaging in regular flexibility exercises aids in muscle recovery by reducing stiffness and soreness, allowing swimmers to maintain consistent training regimens. Furthermore, improved flexibility contributes to a lower risk of overuse injuries, ensuring swimmers can stay in the pool and perform at their best for the long haul.

The Mind-Body Connection:

Beyond the physical benefits, flexibility training nurtures the mind-body connection essential for elite swimmers. Focused stretching sessions provide a mental reprieve, fostering mindfulness and relaxation. This mental resilience translates to heightened focus during races, enabling swimmers to stay in the zone and execute with precision when it matters most.

Incorporating Flexibility into Training:

Integrating flexibility into a swimmer's training regimen doesn't require a complete overhaul. Simple yet effective stretches and yoga poses tailored to the demands of swimming can be seamlessly woven into existing routines. Coaches and swimmers alike should prioritize a holistic approach that balances strength, endurance, and flexibility to maximize overall performance.

Embracing a Culture of Flexibility:

To cultivate a culture of flexibility within the swimming community, coaches play a pivotal role. They should not only advocate for the integration of flexibility exercises but also educate swimmers on the direct correlation between flexibility and performance. Workshops, seminars, or team discussions centered around the importance of flexibility can instill a collective understanding among athletes.

Periodization of Flexibility Training:

Similar to other aspects of a swimmer's training program, flexibility training benefits from a structured periodization approach. This involves varying the intensity and focus of flexibility exercises throughout different phases of the training cycle. Periodization ensures that swimmers continually progress, preventing plateaus and adapting to the specific demands of their competition season.

Cross-Training for Comprehensive Flexibility:

Swimmers can further enhance their flexibility by engaging in cross-training activities that complement their aquatic endeavors. Activities like yoga, Pilates, or even dance can target different muscle groups and movement patterns, contributing to a well-rounded flexibility profile.

Cross-training not only prevents monotony but also introduces novel challenges that promote adaptability and overall physical resilience.

Tracking Progress and Adjusting Flexibility Routines:

Just as swimmers meticulously track their swim times and strength gains, monitoring flexibility progress is equally crucial. Regular assessments, perhaps with the assistance of a certified flexibility coach or physiotherapist, can pinpoint areas that require additional attention. Based on these assessments, coaches can tailor flexibility routines to address individual needs, ensuring a personalized and effective approach to enhancing flexibility.

Yoga Poses to Boost Swimmer's Range of Motion

Downward-Facing Dog (Adho Mukha Svanasana):

stretches the hamstrings, calves, and shoulders.
Strengthens the arms and legs, providing a powerful push-off during swimming starts and turns.

Cobra Pose (Bhujangasana):

Opens the chest and strengthens the back.
Enhances spine flexibility, crucial for maintaining proper body alignment in the water.

Pigeon Pose (Eka Pada Rajakapotasana):

Targets hip flexibility, crucial for powerful kicks and streamlined body positioning.
Alleviates tension in the hips and lower back.

Pose of Threading the Needle (Parsva Balasana):

Releases tension in the shoulders and upper back.

Improves rotational flexibility, essential for efficient strokes like freestyle and backstroke.

Butterfly Pose (Baddha Konasana):

extends the inner thighs and opens the hips.

Enhances the range of motion in the hip joint, promoting a more fluid leg movement in breaststroke.

Bridge Pose (Setu Bandhasana):

hamstrings, glutes, and back are all strengthened.

Boosts flexibility in the spine, promoting a more efficient undulating motion in butterfly strokes.

Extended Triangle Pose (Utthita Trikonasana):

Stretches the sides of the torso, hips, and hamstrings.

Improves lateral flexibility, aiding in smoother side-to-side movements in various strokes.

Bending Forward While Seated (Paschimottanasana):

Lengthens the spine and stretches the hamstrings.

Enhances forward-reaching flexibility, crucial for streamlining the body during dives and turns.

Stretching Sequence for Swimmers

Warm-up:

Begin your stretching routine with a brief warm-up to increase blood flow and prepare your muscles for deeper stretches. Dynamic movements such as arm circles, leg swings, and torso twists are excellent choices to kickstart your flexibility journey.

Neck and Shoulders:

Gentle neck rotations and shoulder rolls help swimmers relieve tension and increase range of motion. These stretches target the upper body, promoting flexibility in crucial areas for efficient stroke execution.

Chest Opener:

Swimming engages the chest muscles significantly. A chest-opening stretch, like clasping your hands behind your back and lifting your arms, counteracts the forward motion of swimming strokes, promoting a balanced upper body.

Spinal Twists:

Improving spinal flexibility is key for swimmers. Incorporate seated or standing spinal twists to enhance rotation, aiding in more efficient turns and reducing strain on the lower back.

Hip Flexor Stretch:

Swimmers rely on powerful kicks, making hip flexibility vital. Incorporate lunges and hip flexor stretches to increase mobility in the hip area, supporting a more streamlined and efficient swimming technique.

Hamstring Stretch:

Flexible hamstrings contribute to a smoother, more powerful kick. Perform seated or standing hamstring stretches to target these muscles, reducing the risk of strain during powerful leg movements.

Quadriceps Stretch:

Maintaining flexibility in the quadriceps is essential for proper leg extension and propulsion. Incorporate standing quad stretches to enhance flexibility in the front thigh muscles.

Calf Stretch:

Powerful ankle flexion is crucial for an effective kick and push-off from walls. Include calf stretches to maintain flexibility in the lower leg, reducing the risk of cramps and improving overall swimming performance.

Finish your stretching sequence with a cooldown to gradually bring your heart rate back to normal and promote flexibility retention. Slow, controlled stretches, combined with deep breathing, will help you relax and reap the full benefits of your stretching routine.

Breathing Techniques for swimmers.

Diaphragmatic Breathing: Dive into the depths with diaphragmatic breathing. Engage your diaphragm to fill your lungs fully, allowing for a more efficient exchange of oxygen and carbon dioxide. This technique not only optimizes oxygen intake but also promotes relaxation, crucial for maintaining composure in challenging swim conditions.

Bilateral Breathing: Achieve balance and symmetry by incorporating bilateral breathing. Alternating sides helps prevent muscle imbalances and enhances overall stroke efficiency. Embrace the cadence of inhaling and exhaling on both sides, creating a fluid and streamlined motion through the water.

Exhalation Timing: Perfect your strokes by synchronizing exhalation with specific phases of your swim. Experiment with exhaling through your nose and mouth during different strokes, discovering the rhythm that complements your individual style. Controlled exhalation aids buoyancy and reduces drag.

Paced Breathing Sets: Elevate your lung capacity with structured breathing sets. Gradually increase breath-holding intervals during training sessions to condition your respiratory system. This method not only strengthens your lungs but also prepares you for controlled breathing in competitive situations.

Open Water Techniques: Conquer the open water with specialized breathing tactics. Practice sighting and breathing simultaneously to maintain course direction without compromising your stroke. Mastering controlled inhalation in challenging environments enhances your adaptability as a swimmer.

Mindful Breathing: Dive into the mindful realm of swimming by focusing on your breath. Cultivate awareness of each inhalation and exhalation, tuning in to the sensations they bring. This mindfulness not only sharpens your concentration but also instills a sense of calm, enhancing your overall swimming experience.

Pre-Race Rituals: Develop pre-race breathing rituals to calm pre-competition nerves. Incorporate deep breaths and positive visualization to create a mental space conducive to peak performance. By mastering the art of pre-race breathing, you set the stage for a confident and composed swim.

Pranayama Exercises to Boost Swimmers' Lung Capacity

Dirga Pranayama, or diaphragmatic breathing:

Begin with the foundation—diaphragmatic breathing. This fundamental pranayama exercise focuses on engaging the diaphragm, allowing swimmers to take fuller, deeper breaths. Practice this on dry land to establish a strong connection between breath and body.

The "Skull-Shining Breath," or Kapalabhati:

Kapalabhati, a dynamic and energizing technique, involves forceful exhalations followed by passive inhalations. This pranayama not only strengthens respiratory muscles but also boosts lung capacity by clearing stale air from the lungs, ensuring a more efficient exchange of oxygen and carbon dioxide.

Ujjayi Pranayama (Victorious Breath):

Known for its calming effects, Ujjayi involves breathing through the nose with a slight constriction at the back of the throat, creating an audible oceanic sound. This controlled breath builds respiratory endurance, helping swimmers maintain a steady rhythm while conserving energy during prolonged swims.

Bhramari (Bee Breath):

Incorporate Bhramari for its soothing impact on the nervous system. By channeling breath through the throat, this pranayama enhances lung capacity and provides swimmers with a valuable tool to manage stress, promoting a focused and composed mindset in challenging swim situations.

Alternative Nostril Breathing, or Nadi Shodhana:

Balance and synchronize the flow of breath with Nadi Shodhana. This pranayama optimizes respiratory function, promoting equal air distribution to both lungs. Swimmers can benefit from improved lung efficiency, translating into enhanced endurance and stamina.

Breathing Routines for Swimmers to Enhance Relaxation and Focus

The Power of Conscious Breathing:

Before the race or training session begins, swimmers can benefit from a few minutes of conscious breathing. Deep, slow breaths activate the parasympathetic nervous system, promoting a sense of calm. This pre-swim ritual establishes a focused mindset, helping swimmers tackle the challenges ahead with composure.

Aligning Breath with Movement:

Incorporating breath control into the stroke rhythm is a game-changer. Aligning inhalations and exhalations with each stroke fosters a harmonious connection between body and breath. This synchronization not only optimizes oxygen intake but also cultivates a rhythmic cadence, enhancing overall swim performance.

Practicing Mindful Breathing Techniques:

Beyond the pool, swimmers can embrace mindfulness through specific breathing techniques. Mindful breathing encourages swimmers to be present in the moment, shedding distractions and honing their concentration. Techniques such as box breathing—inhaling, holding, exhaling, and pausing in equal counts—offer a simple yet potent way to attain mental clarity.

Post-Swim Recovery Breathing:

After a demanding swim session, the importance of post-exercise recovery cannot be overstated. Guided breathing exercises during cool-downs aid in lowering heart rates and easing muscle tension. This deliberate recovery phase contributes to overall well-being and ensures swimmers are ready for their next aquatic endeavor.

Breath Awareness in Water:

Training swimmers to be aware of their breath while submerged adds another layer to their skill set. Controlled breath-holding exercises enhance lung capacity and teach swimmers to navigate underwater environments with confidence. This heightened awareness not only improves technique but also fosters a sense of serenity beneath the water's surface.

The Holistic Impact:

Beyond the physical benefits, incorporating breathing routines into a swimmer's regimen has a holistic impact. Mental resilience, emotional stability, and the ability to navigate high-pressure situations become integral components of a swimmer's toolkit, fostering a well-rounded and adaptable athlete.

The Power of Mind-Body Connection for Swimmers

Harmony in Motion:

Swimming is a dance with the water, and the mind is the choreographer. By cultivating a strong mind-body connection, swimmers synchronize their thoughts with their physical movements. This harmony allows for fluid strokes, improved body awareness, and an enhanced ability to navigate the complexities of different strokes and techniques.

Visualization as a Catalyst:

Picture this: Before you even dive in, mentally visualize the perfect swim. See yourself gliding effortlessly, feel the water's resistance, and imagine the rhythmic breathing. Visualization isn't just a mental exercise; it's a roadmap for your body to follow. As you picture success, your body responds, creating a powerful alignment of intention and action.

Mindful Breathing, Efficient Swimming:

Breathing is the bridge between the mind and body in swimming. Mindful breathing not only optimizes oxygen intake but also serves as a calming force. When swimmers focus on rhythmic and deliberate breathing, they cultivate a serene mental state, ensuring stamina and endurance throughout their laps.

Overcoming Mental Barriers:

Swimming is as much a mental challenge as it is a physical one. The mind-body connection empowers swimmers to break through mental barriers – be it overcoming fear, pushing through fatigue, or staying focused during competition. A resilient mindset transforms challenges into opportunities for growth.

The Flow State:

Ever experience that magical state where everything aligns effortlessly? It's called "flow," and achieving it in swimming requires a seamless mind-body connection. When swimmers enter this state, time seems to slow, movements become instinctive, and peak performance becomes second nature.

Mindfulness Beyond the Pool:

The mind-body connection isn't confined to swim sessions. It permeates daily life, fostering mental resilience and discipline. Swimmers who harness this connection find themselves not just excelling in the pool but navigating life's currents with a calm and purposeful stroke.

The Transformative Power of Meditation for Swimmers

Immersed Tranquility:

Picture the serene calmness beneath the water's edge – a world where distractions fade away. Through meditation, swimmers can tap into this aquatic tranquility, fostering a mindful connection with each stroke and breath.

Focus Amidst the Waves:

The pool's constant ebb and flow mirrors life's challenges. Meditation equips swimmers with the mental fortitude to navigate these waves, fostering unwavering focus amidst the rhythmic chaos of the water.

Breath as the Anchor:

As swimmers delve into meditation, they discover the breath as a reliable anchor. Cultivating conscious breathing not only enhances lung capacity but also becomes a powerful tool for centering the mind, offering respite from the demands of training.

Visualization for Performance:

Through guided meditation, swimmers can visualize their perfect swim – every stroke executed flawlessly, every turn a masterpiece. This mental rehearsal transcends the pool, imprinting a blueprint for success in the subconscious mind.

Stress Dissolved, Performance Elevated:

The demands of competitive swimming can weigh heavily on the mind. Meditation becomes a lifeline, dissolving stress, anxiety, and self-doubt. As mental hurdles crumble, performance soars, unlocking the full potential of every swimmer.

Post-Swim Restoration:

Beyond the pool, meditation aids in the post-swim restoration process. It becomes a ritual for swimmers to unwind, facilitating recovery and promoting a restful state essential for peak performance in subsequent sessions.

Mind-Body Synchronization:

Meditation acts as a bridge between the physicality of swimming and the mental realm. The synchronization of mind and body transforms each swim into a holistic experience, creating a profound connection between the athlete and the water.

The Synergy of Yoga and Swim Training

Fluidity in Motion:

Yoga's emphasis on fluid movements and controlled breathing align seamlessly with the rhythmic strokes of swimming. By incorporating yoga poses that enhance flexibility, such as the Cobra or the Crescent Lunge, swimmers can experience improved range of motion and heightened ease in the water.

Core Strength and Stability:

The core is the epicenter of both yoga and swimming. Poses like Boat Pose or Plank engage and strengthen the core muscles, providing swimmers with enhanced stability and propulsion. A robust core is the key to streamlined swimming and efficient stroke execution.

Mind-Body Connection:

Yoga cultivates a profound mind-body connection, fostering mental clarity and focus. Integrating mindfulness practices into swim training can significantly improve technique and concentration. The serene ambiance of yoga can also serve as a mental retreat, helping swimmers achieve a state of flow during their aquatic endeavors.

Injury Prevention:

Swimmers often face the risk of repetitive stress injuries. Yoga's gentle stretches and poses can alleviate muscular tension, improve joint flexibility, and mitigate the risk of injuries. Incorporating a well-rounded yoga routine into swim training becomes a preventive measure, promoting longevity and sustainability in the water.

Recovery and Relaxation:

The restorative nature of yoga becomes a valuable asset in a swimmer's training regimen. Post-swim yoga sessions aid in muscle recovery, reduce post-exercise soreness, and promote relaxation. The calming effect of yoga complements the invigorating nature of swim training, creating a holistic balance in the overall fitness routine.

Breath Control:

Yoga places a strong emphasis on breath control, an element crucial for swimmers to optimize their respiratory efficiency. Pranayama techniques, like alternate nostril breathing, can be integrated to enhance lung capacity and promote controlled breathing, essential for sustained performance in the water.

Crafting the Perfect Yoga Routine for Swimmers

Pre-Swim Warm-up:

Before hitting the water, indulge in a gentle yoga warm-up. Incorporate sun salutations, dynamic stretches, and controlled breathing to awaken muscles and improve circulation. This primes your body for the aquatic challenge ahead while reducing the risk of injury.

Enhancing Flexibility:

Swimmers often benefit from increased flexibility. Integrate poses like Cobra, Pigeon, and Forward Fold to target key muscle groups, such as the shoulders, hips, and hamstrings. Improved flexibility translates to more efficient strokes and a greater range of motion in the water.

Strength Building for Core Stability:

A strong core is the powerhouse for swimmers. Integrate yoga poses like Boat Pose, Plank, and Warrior III to engage and strengthen your core muscles. This not only enhances stability during swims but also contributes to improved body control and balance.

Breath Control and Lung Capacity:

Yoga places significant emphasis on breath control. Integrate pranayama techniques like Kapalbhati and Ujjayi breathing to enhance lung capacity and control. Improved respiratory function translates to better endurance in the pool, allowing swimmers to maintain optimal oxygen levels during prolonged swims.

Post-Swim Recovery:

After a challenging swim, wind down with yoga poses that promote recovery. Gentle stretches like Child's Pose, Legs Up the Wall, and Corpse Pose help release tension, reduce muscle soreness, and promote relaxation. This aids in quicker recovery and prepares the body for subsequent training sessions.

Mind-Body Connection:

Yoga is renowned for fostering a strong mind-body connection. Incorporate mindfulness practices, such as meditation and visualization, to enhance focus and mental resilience. A calm and focused mind translates to improved performance and enjoyment in the water.

Consistency is Key:

Establishing a consistent yoga routine alongside your swimming regimen is crucial. Aim for a balanced mix of strength, flexibility, and mindfulness practices. Whether it's a short routine before a swim or a dedicated session on rest days, maintaining consistency is key to reaping the full benefits.

Weekly Yoga Schedule for Optimal Results

Monday: Energizing Flow

Kickstart your week with a dynamic, energizing flow that invigorates your body and sharpens your focus. Flow seamlessly through asanas, syncing breath with movement, setting the tone for a vibrant week ahead.

Tuesday: Core Strength and Balance

Engage your core and find your balance as you delve into a session dedicated to building strength from within. Develop a powerful foundation that supports not just your physical practice but also enhances stability in your daily life.

Wednesday: Mindful Meditation

Midweek, immerse yourself in the serenity of mindful meditation. Cultivate mental resilience, reduce stress, and find inner peace as you explore various meditation techniques guided by experienced instructors.

Thursday: Flexibility and Stretch

Unwind midweek with a focus on flexibility and deep stretching. Enhance your range of motion, release tension, and promote flexibility, fostering a sense of ease in both body and mind.

Friday: Restorative Yoga

As the weekend approaches, treat yourself to a restorative yoga session. Rejuvenate your body and mind, allowing gentle poses and mindful breathing to restore balance and prepare you for a rejuvenating weekend.

Saturday: Power Vinyasa

Ignite your inner fire with a powerful Vinyasa flow. Challenge yourself physically and mentally, building strength, endurance, and a profound connection between movement and breath.

Sunday: Yoga Nidra and Reflection

Wrap up your week with a session of Yoga Nidra, a guided meditation that induces deep relaxation. Reflect on your journey, set intentions for the week ahead, and bask in the tranquility that comes with a well-nurtured mind and body.

Benefits of Our Weekly Yoga Schedule

Holistic Wellness: Address physical, mental, and emotional aspects of well-being.

Progressive Growth: Each day complements the others, fostering gradual improvement.

Expert Guidance: Experienced instructors guide you through diverse practices.

Community Support: Join a like-minded community on the path to wellness.

Key Benefits and Takeaways for Swimmers

Physical Fitness Mastery:

Swimming stands as a testament to full-body engagement. The rhythmic strokes and kicks sculpt muscles, enhance cardiovascular health, and contribute to a lean physique. The water's resistance becomes a dynamic gym, fostering strength, endurance, and flexibility in every swimmer.

Mental Resilience Amplified:

Beneath the serene surface, swimmers navigate challenges that require unwavering focus and mental fortitude. The repetitive nature of strokes fosters discipline, concentration, and a resilient mindset – skills that extend beyond the pool into everyday life.

Stress Dissolves in the Water:

Immersing oneself in water is akin to a therapeutic escape. The buoyancy lifts both body and spirit, reducing stress and promoting relaxation. The rhythmic breathing patterns serve as a natural meditation, offering swimmers a sanctuary from the demands of daily life.

Lifelong Social Bonds:

Swimming transcends individual accomplishment; it's a community affair. Whether you're part of a competitive team or a casual swim group, the pool becomes a breeding ground for camaraderie. Shared goals, victories, and even the occasional defeat forge bonds that withstand the test of time.

Life-Saving Skills Unveiled:

Beyond the pursuit of personal records, swimming imparts invaluable life-saving skills. Knowing how to navigate water safely, understanding currents, and mastering various strokes contribute to a heightened sense of water awareness, a skill set that transcends leisure and becomes a life skill.

Time Management Expertise:

Swimmers are masters of the clock, balancing training sessions, competitions, and personal commitments. The discipline required to manage time efficiently in pursuit of aquatic goals spills over into other aspects of life, fostering a well-rounded and organized individual.